HOW TO STOP CHILD ABUSE

Eradicating Abuse on children, preteen and Teenagers

JUDITH WALTER

Copyright©2022: JUDITH WALTER
All RIGHT RESERVED

Table of contents

INTRODUCTION

CHAPTER ONE
- WHAT IS CHILD ABUSE
- CHILD ABUSE TYPE
- CHECKLISTS FOR SEXUAL ABUSE
- CHECKS FOR PHYSICAL ABUSE
- EMOTIONAL ABUSE INDICATORS

CHAPTER TWO
- CHILD ABUSE AND NEGLECT: WHAT ARE THEY?
- HOW MASSIVE IS THE ISSUE?
- POST TRAUMATIC STRESS

CHAPTER THREE
- PERCEIVING CHILD ABUSE

CHAPTER FOUR
- RESULTS OF CHILD ABUSE AND NEGLECT
- NEUROBIOLOGICAL OUTCOMES
- SEPARATION

CHAPTER FIVE
- WELLBEING OUTCOMES
- JUVENILE AND ADULT OUTCOMES
- WRONGDOING AND VIOLENCE

- **LIQUOR AND SUBSTANCE USE**
  <u>CONCLUSION</u>

INTRODUCTION

300 children between the ages of 2 and 4 regularly suffer physical punishment or possible mental violence as a result of guardians and parental figures.

One in five women and one in every thirteen males report having been physically abused as children between the ages of 0 and 17 years.

120 million girls and young women under the age of 20 have engaged in some kind of restricted sexual activity.

Child abuse hurts a child's long-term physical and mental health, and its effects on society and the media may ultimately slow a country's economic and social development.

Savagery is handed down from one generation to the next because a small child who has been mistreated would undoubtedly mistreat others when they are adults. Therefore, it is crucial to end this vicious cycle and produce results that will benefit several generations.

It is possible to stop child abuse before it starts, but this calls for a multisectoral strategy.
Supporting parents, demonstrating loving qualities, and amending laws to forbid harsh punishment are all examples of effective anticipatory strategies.
Taking better care of children and families may diminish the effects of abuse and reduce the likelihood that it will recur.

Child abuse is the mistreatment and disrespect of children under the age of 18. It includes a variety of physical and severe medical treatments, sexual abuse, neglect, negligence, and commercial or another double-dealing that harms or threatens to harm the child's health, resilience, development, or respect in a relationship based on duty, trust, or authority.

WHY DOES IT MATTER?

As they grow older, many children encounter mistreatment of some kind. This may result in fear and alienation feelings. Kid defense administrations (CPS) received 676,000 in the US.

According to one study, one out of every four children will ultimately endure some kind of mistreatment or disrespect. Eyewitnesses may be hesitant to become engaged in the tough subject of child abuse if they are unaware of or have no understanding of what happened in its entirety.

Sometimes people are hesitant to speak out because of the prevailing societal impact. The child may assume that the person manhandling them is overly large or powerful. They can also assume that they won't be welcomed. Additionally, they could feel ashamed, degraded, or stressed out about being at fault.

It might be difficult to spot misuse. Some of the symptoms, such as swelling, may be necessary for normal adolescent development.

Sometimes the abuse is partially the consequence of problems that the parents or other parental figures are having, which also need attention. These could be financial difficulties, unemployment, emotional health problems, or problems with drug abuse. They could have also experienced abuse as children.

Children may benefit from being alerted to warning indications of abnormal behavior, but so might their parents.

CHAPTER ONE
WHAT IS CHILD ABUSE?
Kid abuse goes beyond just physical violence directed at a child. It is any kind of harsh or demeaning abuse committed by an adult against a child. This includes showing disdain.

This is a kind of abusive conduct at home when a child is abused at home and the perpetrator is, for example, the child's parent or guardian.

However, there are times when children are mistreated by other adults that they depend on, such as daycare workers, teachers, and sports coaches.

Misuse may sometimes be intentional but not always. If parents or other parental figures are not yet prepared to change their behavior to concentrate on the child, this may result in inappropriate behavior.

CHILD ABUSE TYPES
There are five main categories of child abuse:

Actual ABUSE includes all forms of cruelty;
Deep or mental abuse: a grownup constantly corrects the child, behaves arrogant and threatening toward the child, or purposely frightens the child.

Actual disregard: The child isn't given the care and assistance it needs.

A constant lack of positive concern for the child may be due to proximity to home or mental disdain. ignoring the child's need for affection, warmth, and security. This course also addresses situations in which children see violence between their parents or other adult family members.

Sexual abuse is when a grownup engages in sexual activity with a child.

TRUE ABUSE

Actual mistreatment may purposefully include:

In many countries, using physical violence toward children for any reason, including punishment, is considered abuse.

devouring or singing suffocating or suffocating, for example, holding a child submerged harming shaking, tossing, hitting, or gnawing without consent extreme squeezing, slapping, or stumbling placing the child in a fixed position while preventing access to rest, food, or drugs Munchausen's condition, also known as a factitious problem foisted on another, is an example of intentionally causing a side effect or encouraging illness in a child (FDAI).
Whipping is becoming seen as a kind of legitimate child abuse in several countries.

CHECKS FOR PHYSICAL ABUSE
The following are symptoms that genuine mistreatment may be taking place, but it's important to remember that they are not proof of mistreatment and might occur for a variety of reasons.
Unaccounted for bruised eyes, broken bones, injuries, chomps or consumes wounds that could reveal an example, such

as multiple consumptions or welts on the hand, dissenting or crying when it's time to enter a specific location, such as a home, school, or another place where abuse could occur having all the telltale signs of being afraid of a specific person being watchful, as though expecting something bad to happen jumping when approached wearing inappropriate clothing

If an adult is engaging in abuse, they might: Use the fear of genuine punishment rather than enforcing rules to regulate a child's mannerisms. Show up too serious and cruel when the child behaves capriciously without logical bounds or regulations. Blow out in wrath when the child does anything wrong.

MENTAL HEALTH TREATMENT

Psychological abuse occurs when people consistently behave and speak in a way that conveys to the child that they are unworthy, unlikeable, ineffective, or just esteemed, all things considered.

This may have a profound, long-lasting impact on the child.

Examples include not allowing children to express their opinions and feelings, mocking what they say, keeping them quiet most of the time, yelling at or undermining them, deriding how they are or how they try to communicate, and giving a child the "quiet treatment" as a form of punishment, restricting actual contact, telling them they are "no decent" or "a slip-up," preventing them from forming typical social connections with friends and other people, and abusing someone else before the child, Psychological maltreatment is a component of many forms of abuse, although it may also occur on its own.

EMOTIONAL ABUSE INDICATES

Some of these symptoms might indicate that a child is being subjected to psychological abuse:

displaying boundaries in behavior, such as consistency, resignation, or forcefulness; seeming distant, restless, or uneasy age-unseemly behavior, such as sucking a thumb, lack of relationship to parent or guardian
abuse of a sexual nature
Sexual abuse is defined as any act that encourages or seduces a child or young person to engage in sexual activity. Regardless of whether the child understands what is happening and if there is power, viciousness, or even touch, it is still sexual abuse.
It is considered sexual abuse if the young person is forced or encouraged to engage in any behavior that stimulates the other.

Such activities might be:
attacks at the door, such as physical or verbal sex, non-penetrative sexual acts, such as touching beyond clothing, scouring, kissing, and stroking off, watching others engage in sexual acts or enticing a child to

do so, looking at, sharing, or discovering sexually explicit images, recordings, toys, or other content, forcing or encouraging a child to strip off for sex, or "blazing" or exposing one's privates to the child
The person who perpetrates the abuse might be an adult male, adult female, or another child, usually, one who has voluntarily reached puberty, but younger children may also abuse.

CHECKLISTS FOR SEXUAL ABUSE
These behaviors in the child might indicate sexual abuse:
looking at being physically abused displaying inappropriate sexual behavior or information that is out of character for their age, odd, or strange withdrawing from friends and family, and leaving the house to avoid a particular person having nightmares or wetting the bed after previously not doing so, changing one's mindset, craving pregnancy, or having an STD that was

physically transmitted, especially before the age of 14 years,
An actual indicator of sexual abuse is having difficulty standing or sitting down.

Usually, someone the child knows is involved in sexual abuse. The child will often admit to keeping the connection a secret. If they inform somebody, they risk having something bad happen that undermines them.

A grownup who abuses a child sexually may have had a similar response in the past. Breaking the loop can help prevent it from happening in the future.

DISREGARD
Misuse may cause forlornness, alienation, and poor confidence, among other long-lasting effects.
Child neglect occurs when a parent or guardian consistently fails to satisfy a child's basic physical and mental needs, posing a

threat to the child's well-being or development.
Parents who are single, in their teens, or who had a bad upbringing may find it challenging.
In certain instances, recognizing parents who need assistance and providing them with assistance and training might help parents prevent abuse while raising their children.

CHAPTER TWO

CHILD ABUSE AND NEGLECT: WHAT ARE THEY?

What are the misuse and disdain of youth? Neglecting children and abusing them are both major medical issues, as are unpleasant youth interactions (ACEs). They have an impact on wealth, opportunity, and well-being. This problem includes a variety of abuse and neglect of a child under the age of 18 by a parent, guardian, or another person in a caring position (such as a strict leader, a mentor, or an educator), which results in harm, the possibility of mischief, or the risk of harm to a child. Four common forms of abuse and disrespect are as follows:

Serious abuse is the willful use of real force that has the potential to cause actual harm. Examples include punching, kicking, shaking, eating, or using other displays of strength against a child.

Sexual abuse comprises pressuring or coercing a child into participating in sexual

acts. It includes actions like cuddling, sneaking around, and exposing a child to other sexual activities. For further information, see the CDC's Preventing Child Sexual Abuse page if it's not too much work. Psychological abuse refers to actions or attitudes that undermine a child's sense of worth or long-term success. Verbal abuse, denigration, dismissal, maintaining love, and undermining are examples.
The inability to satisfy a child's deep and basic needs is disregarded. These prerequisites include things like accommodations, food, clothes, education, admission to clinical consideration, and having one's feelings acknowledged and appropriately addressed.

HOW MASSIVE IS THE ISSUE?
Misuse and disdain by children are common. In the United States, about 1 out of every 7 children has experienced child abuse or neglect in the preceding year. Due to the underreporting of many instances,

this is realistic and undervalued. In 2020, 1,750 children in the United States died as a result of abuse and neglect.

Children who are dependent on others are more likely to be mistreated and ignored. Experiencing impoverishment may be very stressful for families, increasing the risk of child abuse and neglect. Children in low-income homes abuse and ignore adults at rates that are several times higher.

Abuse of children is rampant. In the United States, the total lifetime economic cost of child abuse and neglect was $592 billion in 2018. This financial burden is comparable to the costs associated with other well-known general medical disorders, such as diabetes and cardiovascular disease.

POST TRAUMATIC STRESS
Children who are mistreated and abused may suffer immediate physical injuries including cuts, wounds, or fractured bones.

They could also be dealing with psychological problems that are personal to them, such as stress or posttraumatic stress.

Over time, children who are mistreated or discarded are also more likely to be exposed to future violent crime, drug abuse, physically transmitted infections, postponed mental health, reduced academic success, and constrained professional opportunities.

Constant abuse may result in toxic pressure, which may alter mental health and increase the risk for conditions like posttraumatic stress disorder.
and learning, consideration, and memory troubles.
How might we forestall youngsters' misuse and disregard?
Youngster misuse and disregard are preventable. Certain elements might increment or abate the gamble of executing or encountering kid misuse and disregard. To forestall youngsters' misuse and

disregard of viciousness, we should comprehend and address the variables that put individuals in danger or shield them from brutality. Everybody benefits when youngsters have protected, stable, supporting connections and conditions. CDC created Preventing Child Abuse and Neglect: A Technical Package for Policy, Norm, and Programmatic Activities pdf icon to assist networks with utilizing the most ideal that anyone could hope to find proof to forestall kid misuse and disregard. This asset is accessible in English and Spanish pdf icons and can affect individual ways of behaving and connections, family, local area, and cultural elements that impact risk and defensive variables for youngsters misuse and disregard.

Various kinds of viciousness are associated and frequently share underlying drivers. Kid misuse and disregard are connected to different types of viciousness through shared risk and defensive variables. Tending to and forestalling one type of viciousness might affect forestalling different types of savagery.

CHAPTER THREE

PERCEIVING CHILD ABUSE

Youngster misuse alludes to any close-to-home, sexual, or actual abuse or disregard by a grown-up in a job of liability toward somebody who is under 18 years old. It alludes to any sort of activity or inability to act that results in mischief or conceivable damage to a youngster. The grown-up might be a parent or other relative or another guardian, including sports mentors, instructors, etc.

The Centers for Disease Control and Prevention (CDC) characterize the sorts of believed wellsprings of kid maltreatment as actual maltreatment, sexual maltreatment, psychological mistreatment, or disregard. Misuse frequently includes at least one of these sorts. Tormenting is excluded from these classes, however, it is an approach to conveying various types of misuse.

The activity might be fierce.

It can occur at home or somewhere else, and it happens in all societies, nations, and financial classes. It for the most part includes a relative or companion, instead of an outsider.

It can likewise occur for various reasons, for instance, emotional well-being issues influencing the individual who conveys the maltreatment.

The sorts of misuse that they include and a few signs to pay special attention to.

Quick realities on kid misuse
Four sorts of misuse are disregard and physical, profound, and sexual maltreatment.
In certain nations, utilizing flogging is viewed as youngster misuse.
Indications of misuse can be difficult to identify, yet being removed, detached, and excessively agreeable might be a sign.

The individual who is completing the maltreatment may likewise require help, for instance, a focus on the parent.

Would it be Advisable for me to REPORT THIS?
Kids might communicate their encounters through drawings or play.
A person who thinks or accepts a kid is encountering misuse ought to make a move, for the youngster's prompt and long-haul wellbeing. You needn't bother with to be certain maltreatment is happening or to realize which type.
In the long haul, misuse can prompt issues with trust and relationship hardships, a sensation of uselessness, and trouble controlling feelings. At times, the youngster might develop into a grown-up who manhandles kids in their consideration.

If it is your kid, you ought to eliminate the kid from the individual's presence, for instance, by dropping a sitter for a brief time or potentially for all time, assuming that fears give off an impression of being grounded.

One sign that might show that misuse has occurred is kids causing drawings that address their experience or carrying on what has befallen them in play.
Specialists have said there is an absence of goal estimates that can be utilized to affirm the utilization of drawings as proof for use in a lawful case. Notwithstanding, if a youngster draws uncommon pictures, these might be worth consideration, particularly assuming there are different signs.

No two cases must be something very similar. The signs, as well, may cover. Forceful conduct changes, for instance, could be an indication of either physical or psychological mistreatment.

What's more, different variables can set off comparable side effects. The passing of a friend or family member, partition, or separation, in addition to other things, can likewise cause indications of profound pressure.

Kids who might have encountered misuse ought to visit a specialist or emergency clinic, as actual clinical assistance or guidance might be required.

Anybody who accepts they are manhandling, have mishandled, or could mishandle a kid ought to eliminate themselves from the youngster and spot the kid someplace protected, for instance, by asking another person to care for them, then track down somebody to trust in. Guiding might be essential.

There are helplines accessible, and the nearby police or wellbeing administrations can help. Calls can be made namelessly. The fitting individuals will make a move to explore.

Ways to lessen the gamble
Conversing with youngsters can raise their mindfulness and set them up to perceive and potentially keep away from future issues.
conversing with your youngster about fitting and improper ways of behaving and protected and dangerous circumstances pretending what to do if at any time somebody acts improperly, and how to find support
empowering open correspondence with your youngster, as this will make it more straightforward to detect if anything surprising occurs
guarantee that your own home and yard are protected and plan to ensure you never need to let small kids be
continuously knowing where your youngster is the point at which they are out
Building associations with individuals who take care of your youngsters, including educators, sitters, and guardians of

companions, can help in more ways than one.

It makes it more straightforward to lay out rules for well-being and the proper way of behaving, for instance, what to do if a youngster gets out of hand. It might help distinguish and forestall conceivable maltreatment. It likewise assists fabricate a local area around your youngster that with canning offers extra help and watchfulness.

CHAPTER FOUR
RESULTS OF CHILD ABUSE AND NEGLECT

Sensational advances have been made in understanding the causes and results of youngster misuse and disregard, remembering progresses for the brain, genomic, conduct, psychologic, and sociologies. These advances have started to illuminate logical writing, offering new bits of knowledge into the brain and natural cycles related to youngsters' misuse and disregard and at times, revealing insight into the components that intercede the social sequelae that describe kids who have been manhandled and dismissed. Research additionally has extended how we might interpret the physical and social wellbeing, scholarly, and financial results of youngster misuse and disregard. Information on delicate periods — the possibility that for those parts of mental health that are reliant upon experience, there are stages in which the typical course of advancement is additional helpless to disturbance from experiential irritations — likewise has expanded dramatically. Also, research has started to investigate contrasts in individual defenselessness to the unfavorable results related to youngster misuse and disregard and to reveal the elements that safeguard some c experienced are more inconvenient because a review of kid misuse and disregard can be impacted by various factors and open to various possible predispositions. Aftereffects of studies in light of treatment tests of grown-ups who experienced abuse as youngsters might be possibly one-sided because not all survivors of kid misuse and disregard look for treatment as grown-ups, and because individuals who in all actuality do look for treatment might have higher paces of issues than individuals who don't look for treatment. At the point when members are approached to investigate conditions, for example, current sorrow and history of youngster misuse and disregard, the additional issue of shared technique fluctuation emerges. Then again, utilization of true records raises the issue of underreporting.

The central government has upheld a work, sent off since the 1993 NRC report was given — the National Survey of Child and Adolescent Well-Being (NSCAW) — to extend comprehension of the results of youngster misuse and disregard. This study incorporates the utilization of different information sources and record audits, as well as meetings with kids and youth who have encountered youngster misuse and disregard, their overseers, and kid government assistance laborers.

This part contains a broad audit of the later organically based investigations of youngster misuse and disregard as a result of the significant advances that have been made around here. To the degree conceivable, the conversation depends on discoveries by concentrating on describing the best systemic meticulousness.

Regardless of ongoing strategic advances, scientists face many provokes in endeavoring to comprehend the short-and long haul results of the different sorts of youngster misuse and disregard (e.g., actual maltreatment, sexual maltreatment, disregard from guardians) for a kid working and improvement. One of those difficulties is prodding separating the effect of youngster misuse and disregard from that of other co-happening factors.

For instance, youngsters engaged with kid defensive administrations due to disregard or manhandling frequently face various covering and simultaneous gambling factors, including destitution, pre-birth substance openness, and parent psychopathology, among others. These simultaneous gamble variables can make it especially hard to draw causal inductions about the particular results of misuse and disregard for kids' work, however, should be unraveled from the particular impacts of misuse and disregard. Controlling for other important factors becomes imperative since the inability to consider such family factors might bring about detailing fake connections. A few investigations consider and cover other gamble variables, and some don't. Taking into account the course of misuse and disregard may likewise be especially significant, as Jonson-Reid and partners (2012) found that the quantity of youngster misuse and disregard reports effectively anticipated unfriendly results across a scope of spaces.

Finding: Risk factors that co-occur with youngster misuse and disregards, like destitution, pre-birth substance openness, and parent psychopathology, can bewilder endeavors to draw causal inductions about the particular results of misuse and disregard for kids' working. These elements should be controlled for in examinations looking to recognize the particular results of kid misuse and disregard.

NEUROBIOLOGICAL OUTCOMES

A satisfactory parental figure is expected to help create cerebrum engineering and the ability to control conduct, feelings, and physiology for small kids. At the point when kids experience misuse or disregard, such advancement can be compromised. The impacts of misuse and disregard are seen particularly in cerebrum locales that are subject to natural contribution for the ideal turn of events, and on parts of working particularly vulnerable to ecological info. Right off the bat being developed, babies are dependent on input from their guardians for help in directing excitement, neuroendocrine working, temperature, and other essential capabilities. With time and with effective encounters in co-guideline, youngsters progressively assume control over these capabilities themselves. Misuse and disregard address the shortfall of satisfactory contribution (as on account of disregard) or the presence of undermining input (as on account of misuse), both of which can think twice about. The accompanying segments present a survey of proof for key neurobiological frameworks that are modified because of misuse and disregard right off the bat throughout everyday life: the hypothalamic-pituitary-adrenal (HPA) hub of the pressure reaction framework; the amygdala, engaged with feeling handling and feeling guideline; the hippocampus, engaged with learning and memory; the corpus callosum, engaged with coordinating capabilities among halves of the globe; and the prefrontal cortex, associated with higher-request mental capabilities. The conversation starts, nonetheless, with a short outline of mental health.

Outline of Neurobiological Development
The Construction of the Brain
Mental health starts only half a month after origination, beginning with the development of the brain tube. This is trailed by the age of

various classes of synapses — neurons and glia. When framed, these juvenile neurons start their transitory stage (by and large away from the ventricular zone, which is their starting place) to construct the cerebral cortex. A lot of cell relocation is finished before the second's over trimester of pregnancy, at last prompting the development of the six-layered cerebral cortex. After these youthful cells have moved to their objective, they can separate; that is, they foster cell bodies and cycles (axons and dendrites). Whenever processes have been shaped, neurotransmitters start to frame; neural connections are the associations between neurons that take into consideration the transmission of signs across the synaptic parted, which is the little space that exists between two contiguous synapses, by and large between a dendrite and an axon. The neurotransmitter grants one neuron to speak with another, and ultimately, whole circuits are fabricated, trailed by brain organizations (i.e., coordinated units). At long last, a few axons in the cerebrum foster a covering called myelin that speeds the progression of data along the length of the axon. Tangible pathways start to myelinate during the last trimester of pregnancy, though the affiliation region of the mind, especially the prefrontal cortex, proceeds to myelinate through the second ten years of life. Brain components (e.g., axons) that are covered with myelin are alluded to as white matter, while the greater part of the remainder of the cerebrum is alluded to as dim matter. Numerous parts of mental health (especially those that happen before birth) fall under hereditary control (albeit some are impacted by experience — pre-birth openness to neurotoxins, for example, liquor being nevertheless one model). After birth, notwithstanding, quite a bit of mental health becomes subject to encounter. For instance, albeit the age of neurotransmitters — which are enormously overproduced right off the bat being developed — is generally under hereditary control, the pruning of neural connections — which happens fundamentally after birth — is to a great extent under experiential control. Accordingly, the prefrontal cortex of the 1-year-old youngster has a lot larger number of neurotransmitters than the grown-up cerebrum, however throughout the following one to twenty years, these neural connections are pruned back to grown-up numbers, dependent to a great extent upon experience.

Brain Plasticity and Sensitive Periods

Numerous parts of mental health rely upon encounters happening during specific periods, frequently the initial not many long periods of life. These alleged delicate or basic periods address essential expression focuses throughout improvement, to such an extent that assuming explicit encounters neglect to happen inside some restricted window of time (or some unacceptable encounters happen), advancement can turn out badly. This prompts the idea that pliancy "cuts the two different ways," intending that assuming the kid is presented with great encounters, the cerebrum benefits, however assuming the youngster is presented with awful encounters or insufficient info, the mind might endure. Prenatally, an illustration of a terrible encounter is openness to neurotoxins like liquor or medication misuse. An illustration of a decent encounter is admittance to great sustenance, including the numerous micronutrients that work with mental health (e.g., iron, zinc). Postnatally, the subject of this report addresses instances of awful insight (i.e., misuse and disregard). On the other hand, instances of good encounters incorporate giving a youngster steady, delicate providing care; a sustaining home overall; and sufficient feeling.

As a general rule, most tangible frameworks foster right off the bat throughout everyday life; hence the capacity to see and to separate and perceive countenances and discourse sounds come on line in the principal long periods of life, in light of suitable encounters happening during that time window (e.g., openness to faces, to discourse). This isn't shocking given the way that fundamentally significant these capabilities are to the ensuing turn of events (e.g., language isn't learned until youngsters can separate the essential units of sound, for example, one consonant from another). Basic to the conversation in this section, in any case, is that the capabilities supported by a few different locales of the cerebrum, most quite the prefrontal cortex — leader control, arranging, mental adaptability, feeling guidelines — have a significantly more extended course of improvement for the straightforward explanation that both synaptogenesis and myelination of these cortical districts don't develop until mid-to-late pre-adulthood, maybe even a piece later. Thus, the delicate period for prefrontal cortical capabilities might be more drawn out than is the situation for tangible capabilities, broadening greatly into the young adult time frame. One illustration of the differential time course of various brain

Oppositional defiant disorder and conduct disorder Review have detailed critical relationships between a past filled with youth misuse or disregard and different lead issues, including those named oppositional rebellious turmoil or direct problem. Oppositional insubordinate turmoil is demonstrated by a successive or tenacious example of a furious or crabby mindset, contentious or resistant way of behaving, and malevolence. Its side effects normally first show up during youth, and it frequently goes before direct turmoil, uneasiness issues, or significant burdensome problems. Direct confusion is shown by a dull or determined example of conduct that disregards the fundamental freedoms of others or major cultural standards or rules, including hostility toward individuals or creatures, obliteration of property, underhandedness or burglary, and serious infringement of rules. Direct confusion can start in youth or pre-adulthood; be that as it may, adolescence's beginning behavior problem is all the more frequently gone before by oppositional disobedient turmoil, more tireless into adulthood, and bound to incorporate a forceful way of behaving than puberty beginning behavior issue.

SEPARATION

Separation is characterized as a "disturbance of as well as brokenness in the typical, emotional coordination of at least one part of mental working, including — however not restricted to — memory, character, cognizance, discernment, and engine control" Separation can be estimated dependably and legitimately in kids, young people, and grown-ups. Youngster misuse and disregard have been related to o separation among both preschool-matured and rudimentary matured kids as well as among grown-ups The presence of a subgroup of PTSD patients with elevated degrees of separation has been exhibited in clinical psychophysiological, neuroimaging, and epidemiological research. Subsequently, DSM-V is adding a dissociative subtype to the PTSD determination.

High scores on separation measures have shown to be an indicator of externalizing conduct in youngsters. In grown-ups, elevated degrees of separation are related to stubbornness to standard medicines for various mental circumstances, as well as expanded comorbidity.

A meta-examination of 55 investigations joins maltreatment with a muddled connection. found that moms who participated in disturbed full of feeling correspondence with their newborn children at 4 months (as estimated utilizing the AMBIANCE scale) were bound to have babies who were delegated disarranged at 14 months. Thus, disarranged connection at 14 months anticipated high separation scores at age 20 years. Complicated connections

surveyed during the youngster's subsequent year anticipated raised degrees of self-revealed separation in mid-puberty (age 16 years) and early adulthood (age 19).
In light of discoveries from the Minnesota Mother-Child Project, Egeland and Susman suggest that separation might go about as a go-between of kid maltreatment across ages. In a longitudinal investigation of physically manhandled young ladies followed into life as a parent, Kim and partners found that expanded separation, along with a background marked by self-revealed correctional nurturing as a kid, anticipated whether a mother would parent her kids in a cruel and reformatory way. Hence, a speculative generational circle can be guessed in which brutal and oppressive nurturing builds the gamble for more elevated levels of separation in youth and puberty, which thus expands the gamble for rash ways of behaving and unforgiving nurturing of posterity. Further examination, particularly with a longitudinal plan, is

justified to decide if this conjectured generational example of transmission addresses an early chance for counteraction of maltreatment in the future.

Finding: because of oppressive or careless reactions from guardians, youngsters struggle with creating coordinated and secure connections. Subsequently, mishandled and ignored youngsters are at a higher gamble for the improvement of relational issues, especially disinhibited social commitment problems.

Finding: Abused and disregarded youngsters frequently neglect to foster powerful techniques for feeling guidelines, halfway because of contrasts in the handling of close-to-home signals. Hardships with feeling guidelines can prompt further issues, including externalizing and assimilating issues and difficulties in peer relations.

Finding: Children who experience misuse or disregard have been viewed as at a higher gamble for the advancement of externalizing conduct issues, including oppositional resistant confusion, lead jumble, and forceful ways of behaving. Manhandled and ignored kids likewise have been viewed as at expanded risk for incorporating issues, especially sorrow, in youth, immaturity, and adulthood.

Finding: Among preschool-and primary school-matured youngsters, as well as grown-ups, a background marked by youth misuse and disregard has been related to separation, which builds the gamble for externalizing conduct in adolescence and protection from treatment for mental circumstances sometime down the road. It has been recommended that separation might go about as a middle person of unforgiving or oppressive nurturing across ages, albeit this theory requires further exploration.

Finding: various investigations have tracked down raised paces of PTSD among people with a background marked by misuse and disregard. PTSD has been related to physical, mental, mental, social, and conduct issues among youth who were manhandled or ignored in adolescence.

CHAPTER FIVE

WELLBEING OUTCOMES

Kid misuse and disregard significantly affect various well-being results, from development to disease to weight. Associations have been found between hazardous neurobiological results of kid misuse and disregard and wellbeing. One conceivable instrument for these impacts connects with the indicated successive or ongoing enactment of the HPA hub. As talked about beforehand, the HPA hub is intended for answering in emergencies.

JUVENILE AND ADULT OUTCOMES

While some of the results of kid misuse and disregard examined already in this part can be available across youth, puberty, and adulthood, this segment centers around social results that manifest explicitly in one or the other pre-adulthood or adulthood.

WRONGDOING AND VIOLENCE

Misuse and disregard experienced in youth anticipated savagery and captures in early adulthood. Grown-ups with a background marked by misuse and disregard were more probable than grown-ups without such a set of experiences to have perpetrated non traffic offenses (49% versus 38%) and brutal wrongdoings (18% versus 14%). Survivors of young life actual maltreatment and disregard were bound to be captured for brutality (chances proportions 1.9 and 1.6, individually) after controlling for age, race, and sex. These creators additionally observed that manhandled and dismissed young ladies were at expanded risk of being captured for viciousness compared with young ladies who had not been mishandled and ignored, with a chances proportion of 1.9. Smith and partners (2005) likewise found that maltreatment and disregard increment the gamble of rough culpable in late puberty and early adulthood.

Jonson-Reid and partners (2012) found a strong impact on the quantity of kid misuse reports anticipating brutal wrongdoing, with the affiliation being direct for up to three reports. Two of these imminent longitudinal investigations additionally discovered that sexual maltreatment expanded the gamble for general culpable, however not vicious culpable. Actual maltreatment gives off an impression of being firmly connected with viciousness in young ladies, as exhibited in a meta-examination.

There is proof that youth misuse expands the gamble for wrongdoing and misconduct. Various huge forthcoming examinations in various parts of the United States have reported a connection between youth misuse and disregard and adolescent as well as youthful grown-up wrongdoing.

Notwithstanding contrasts in a geographic area, period, young people's age and sex, the meaning of kid abuse, and evaluation method, these imminent examinations give proof that youth abuse increments later gamble for wrongdoing and brutality. Replication of this relationship across various very much planned examinations upholds the generalizability of and increments trust in the outcomes.

LIQUOR AND SUBSTANCE USE

As teenagers and grown-ups, those with a background marked by misuse and disregard have higher rates of liquor misuse and liquor abuse than those without a background marked by misuse and disregard. The impacts will quite often be more grounded for ladies, being seen in any event, when different elements are covered. For instance, Winny and her partners found no relationship between a background marked by misuse and disregard and liquor use by young fellows, yet found a relationship for ladies even after controlling for parental substance use and other corresponded factors. A comparable example of results arose in development with these members around 10 years after the fact, when they were roughly 40 years of age. Ladies with a reported history of kid misuse as well as disregard were bound to drink unreasonably in center adulthood than those without such a set of experiences once more, this distinction was not found in men. Young ladies with a background marked by actual maltreatment will more often than not begin utilizing substances The find

Ten steps you can do to stop child abuse
Give of your time. Join forces with other parents in your neighborhood. Help the families and vulnerable children. Start a playgroup.

Mindfully discipline your kids. Never give your kid a punishment while you are angry. Give yourself some time to relax. Do not forget that discipline is a method of teaching your kid. You may help your youngster recover control by using time-outs and privileges to reward appropriate conduct. Analyze your actions. Abuse extends beyond the physical. Deep, long-lasting wounds may be caused by both words and deeds. Be a devoted parent. Show youngsters and other adults via your actions that disputes can be resolved without violence or screaming. Teach others and yourself. The simplest strategy to stop child abuse may be to provide simple assistance for kids and parents. Children may be protected from violence in a variety of ways, including via after-school activities, parent education workshops, mentorship programs, and respite care. Be an advocate for these initiatives in your neighborhood.

Educate kids about their rights. Children are less likely to believe that abuse is their fault and more willing to report a perpetrator when they are taught that they are unique and have a right to safety.

Encourage preventative initiatives. Intervention happens all too often after the abuse has been reported. Increased funding is required for initiatives that have been shown to prevent abuse before it starts, such as family counseling and nurse home visits that help parents and babies.

Identify child maltreatment. Maltreatment includes both physical and sexual abuse, but it also includes neglect, which is when parents or other caretakers fail to provide a kid with the necessary care, food, and clothes. When children are repeatedly isolated, rejected, or reprimanded, this may also constitute emotional abuse against them.

Recognize the symptoms; abuse may manifest itself in a variety of ways. Depression, anxiety about a particular adult, lack of social skills or trust in others, abrupt changes in eating or sleeping habits, inappropriate sexual behavior, poor hygiene, secrecy, and hostility are frequent indicators of family issues and may be signs of neglect or physical, sexual, or emotional abuse of a child.

Report any abuse. Report any suspected or actual child abuse to your state's child protective services agency or the local police if you observe it happening. When discussing the abuse with a kid, pay close attention, reassure the child that reporting the abuse to an adult was the correct thing to do, and reaffirm that the child is not to blame for what occurred.

Invest in children. Encourage local authorities to help young people and families. Ask companies to provide workplaces that are accommodating to families. Ask your local and federal officials to support legislation that would enhance and better safeguard the lives of our children.

CONCLUSION

PROTECTING YOUR KID FROM HARM

Your first defense against child abuse may be as simple as talking to your kid. If you establish an honest and trustworthy connection with your kid, you are more likely to identify any danger to their safety. Some phrases you may use to keep your kid secure

You should discuss the following topics with your child:

1. Reassure your kid that they will not suffer consequences if they report feeling unsafe or intimidated in any manner by anybody. Your child has a right to safety (including family members)

2 Encourage your kid to tell you if something is making them feel uneasy, perplexed, or afraid. The truth will always be believed (children rarely lie about abuse)

3.Talk to your kid about the parts that should be covered (swimsuit regions) and urge them to let you know if someone attempts to go beyond these limits since their body is their own.

4.say 'no' - Children often believe that they must follow adult instructions, especially if they have been forced to hug or kiss adults against their will since abusers and bullies sometimes claim that their actions are "our secret" or even jeopardize the safety of other family members. Tell your youngster that keeping secrets like that is never a good idea.

5.Assure your kid that reporting abuse would not cause any damage to them or their loved ones.

If a stranger approaches your kid, instruct them to ignore them and run to you right away.

These latter two points apply to a variety of circumstances:

6.Encourage your kid to shout, kick, scream, lie, or run away if they believe they are in danger by telling them it is appropriate to disobey the rules in an emergency.
Have a secret phrase or sign that you and your kid (as well as another parent or caretaker) may use to retrieve your child if necessary.

7.Children must understand that they are unique, cherished, and capable of pursuing their aspirations.
Support a friend, neighbor, or family member.

8.Parenting is not simple. Put a helping hand in it and look after the kids so the parents may relax or enjoy time together. Assisted by you.

9.Take a break when your daily concerns, both large and little, overwhelm you and make you feel out of control. Don't lash out at your child.

If your infant wails,

10. Being frustrated by your baby's crying is normal. Find out what to do if your child won't stop sobbing. Never shake a baby; doing so might cause serious harm or even death.
Get active.
11. Ask your local authorities, church, libraries, and schools to provide services that cater to the needs of happy families and healthy children.

12. Participate in creating parenting materials at your neighborhood library. Check to see whether your local library provides parenting materials and if not, volunteer to help find some.

13. Promote school initiatives.
Children may be kept safe by being taught preventative techniques by parents, teachers, and other caregivers.

14. Keep an eye on your child's use of the internet, video, and television.
The excessive viewing of violent movies, TV shows, and videos might be harmful to young children.

 cause to suspect a kid has been or may be harmed.